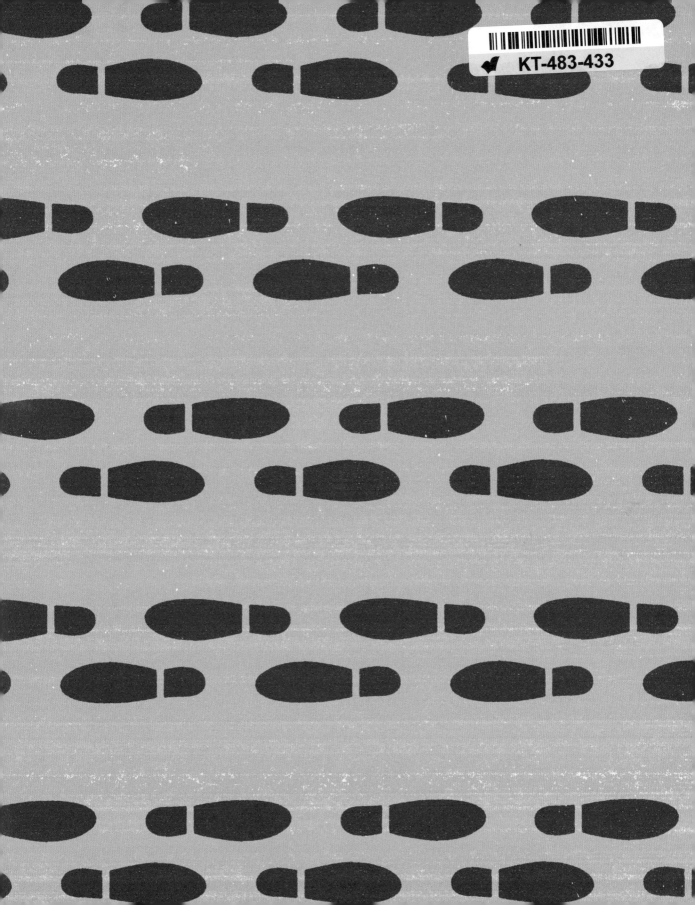

Little People, BIG DREAMS®
CAPTAIN TOM

Written by
Maria Isabel Sánchez Vegara

Illustrated by
Christophe Jacques

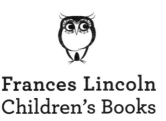

Frances Lincoln
Children's Books

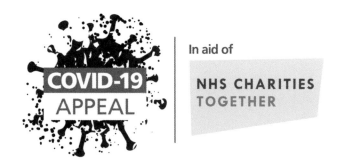

Little People, BIG DREAMS®
CAPTAIN TOM

Written by
Maria Isabel Sánchez Vegara

Illustrated by
Christophe Jacques

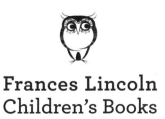

Frances Lincoln
Children's Books

Once there was a humble boy from Yorkshire who was born with his feet firmly on the ground.

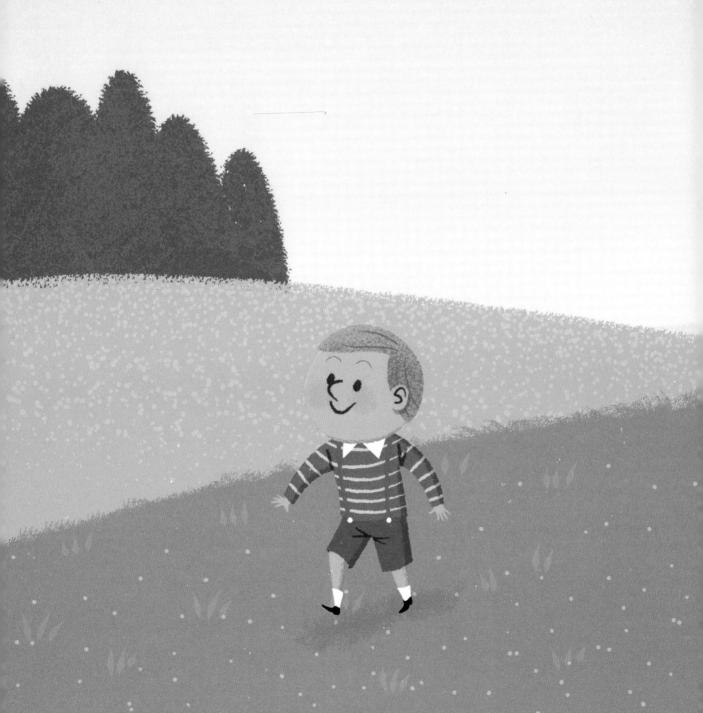

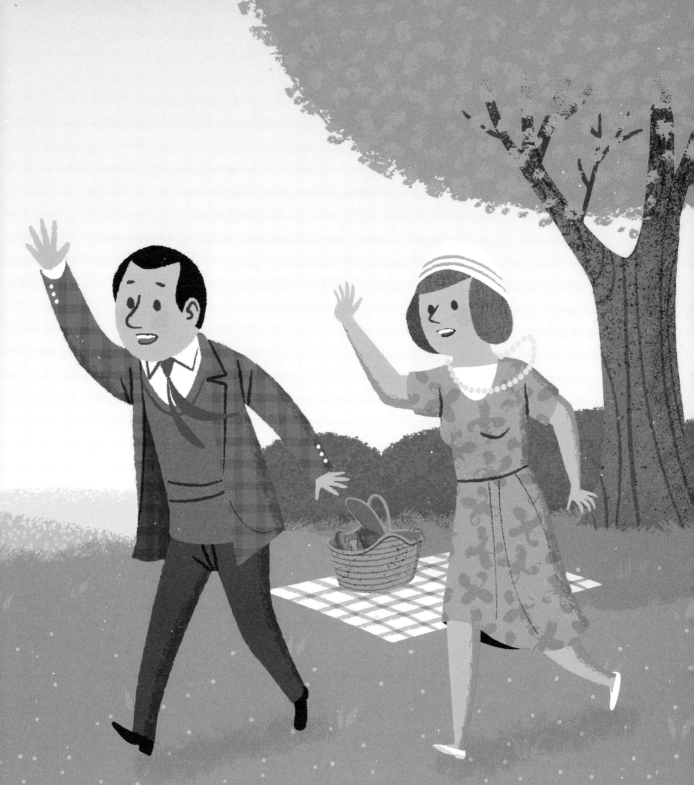

His name was Tom, and the day he started
walking his parents realised he would never stop.

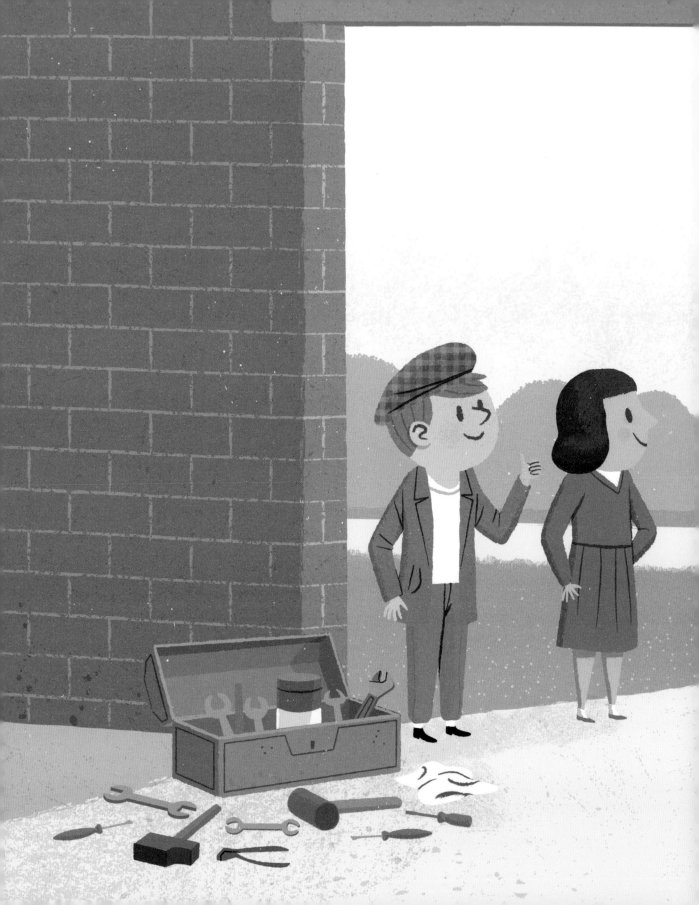

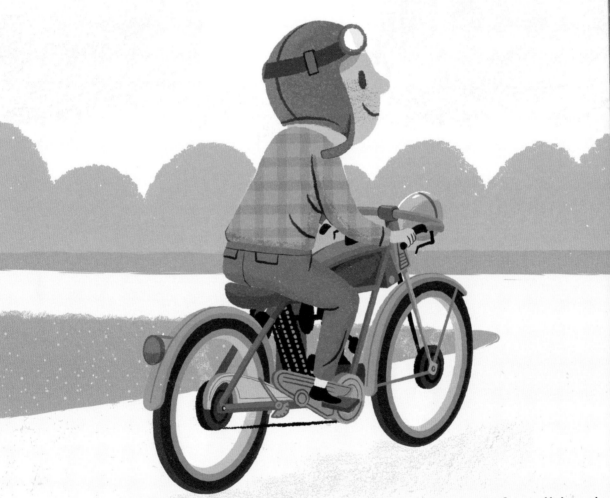

From an early age, he showed a passion for all kinds of engines. Tom was just twelve when he found a broken motorcycle in a barn. He bought it for two shillings and sixpence, determined to fix it and take to the road.

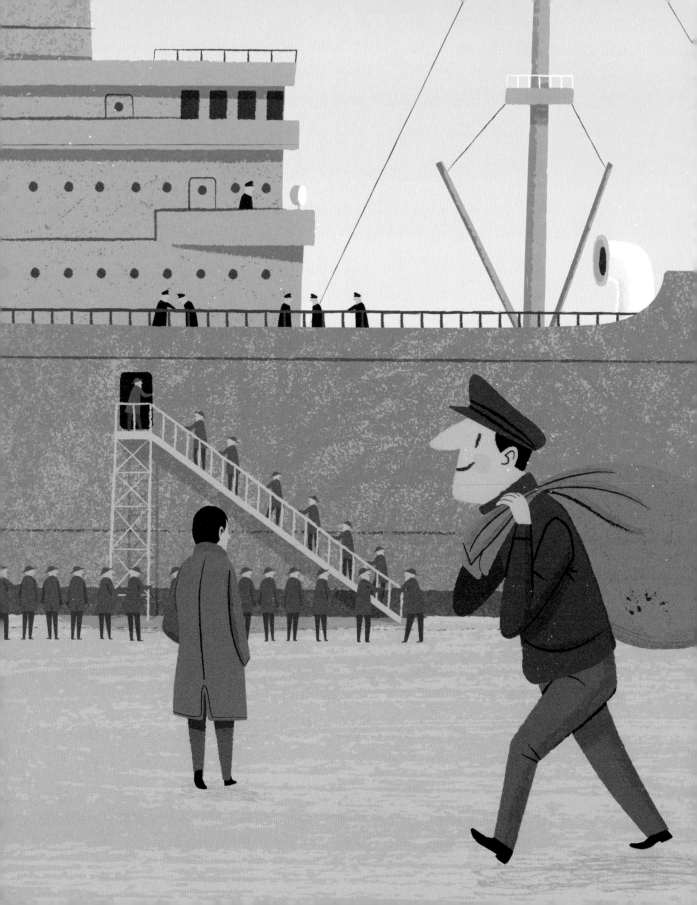

Tom was working as an apprentice engineer when he was called up to join the Duke of Wellington's Regiment and fight for his country in a faraway land. He had never left his family before, but his knees did not tremble.

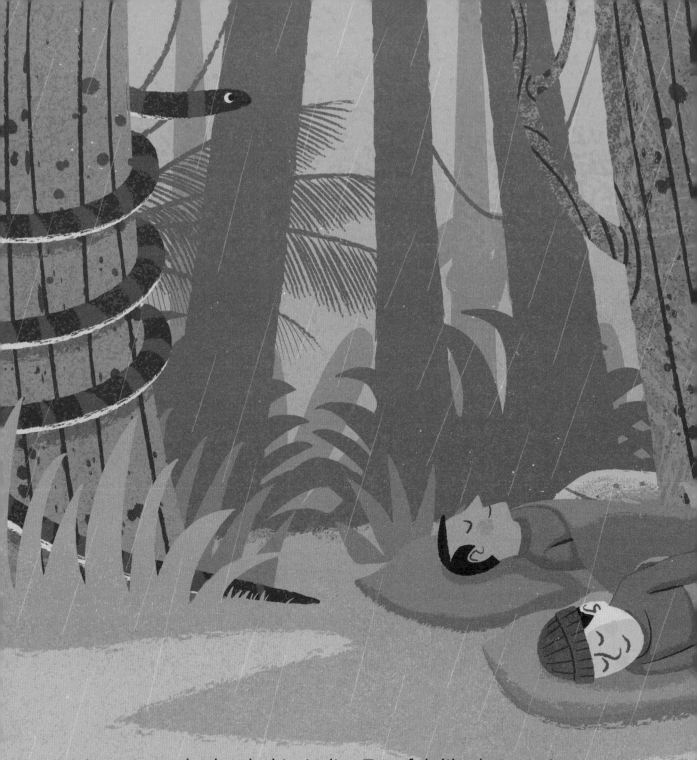

As soon as he landed in India, Tom felt like he was in an entirely new world. Sometimes, he had to share his bed with spiders as big as the palm of his hand, and poisonous snakes, but next to his comrades he felt at home.

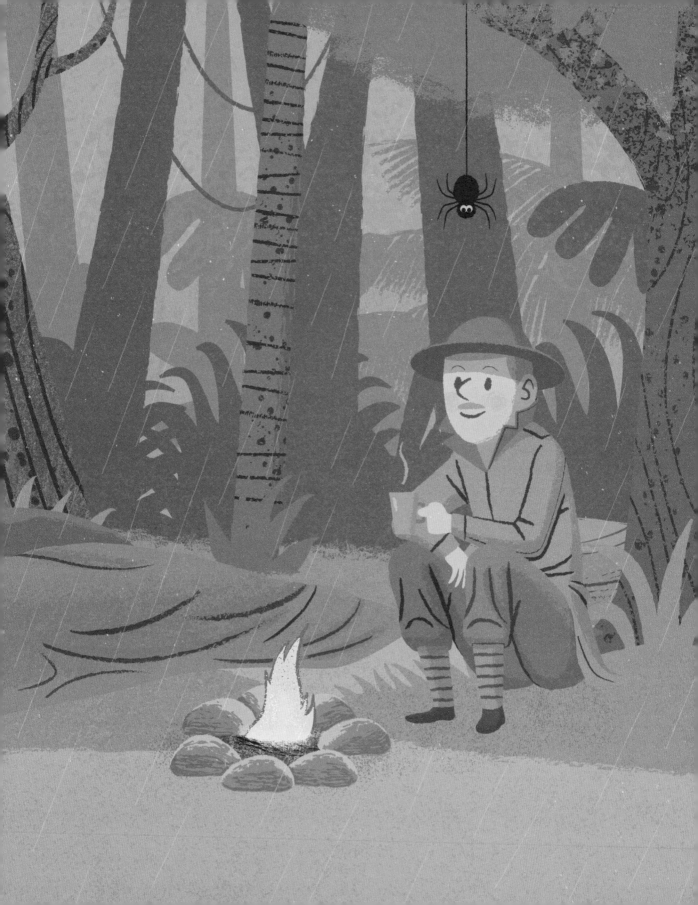

His firm determination and courage took him from soldier to Captain. Tom was always there to raise his team's spirits. Even in their toughest moments, under enemy fire, he knew they were on the winning side.

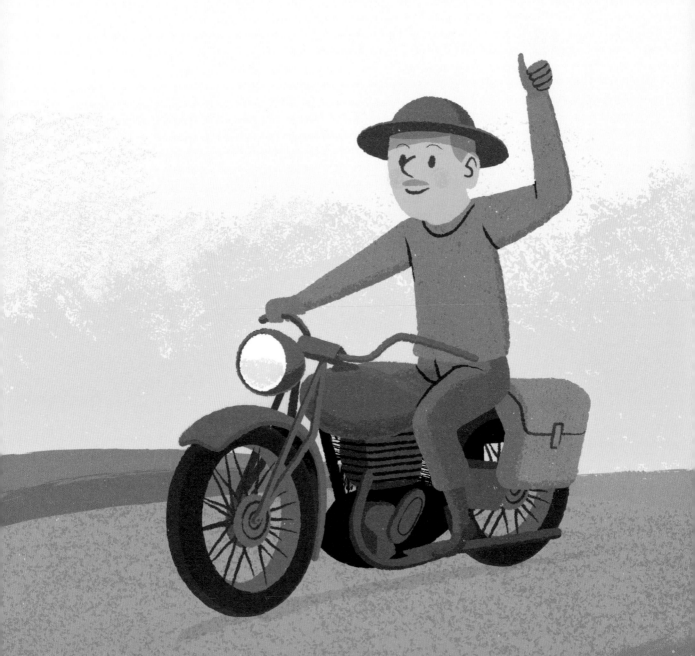

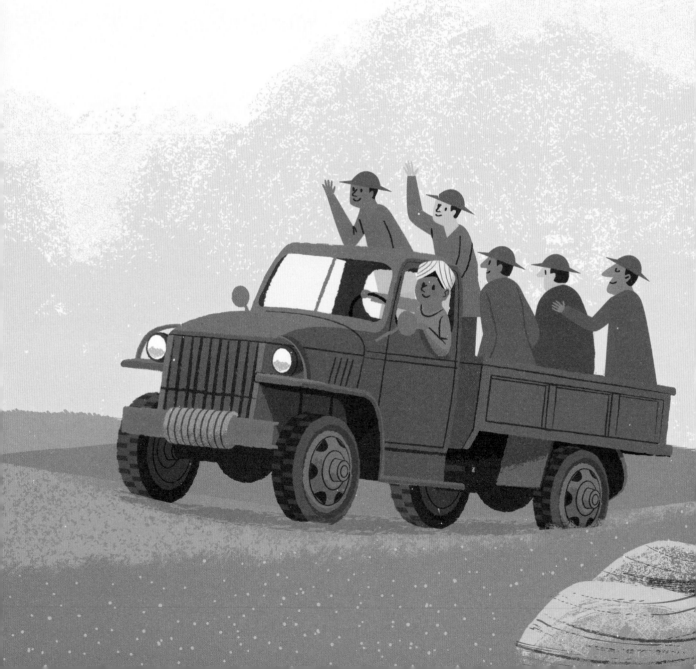

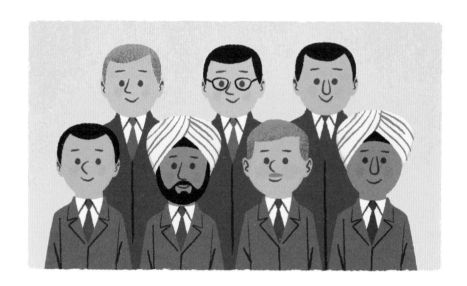

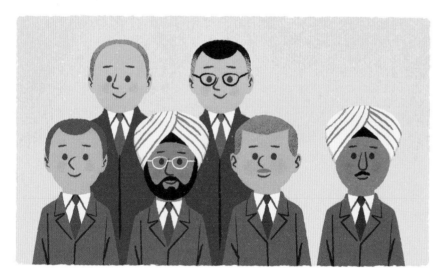

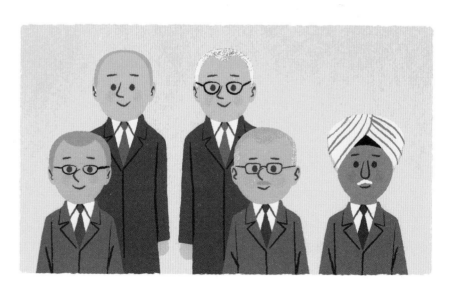

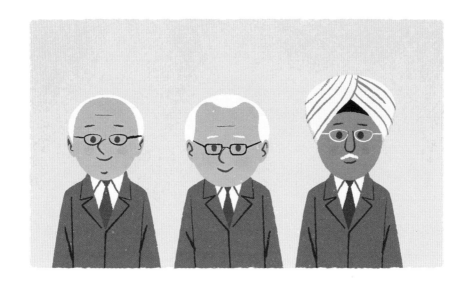

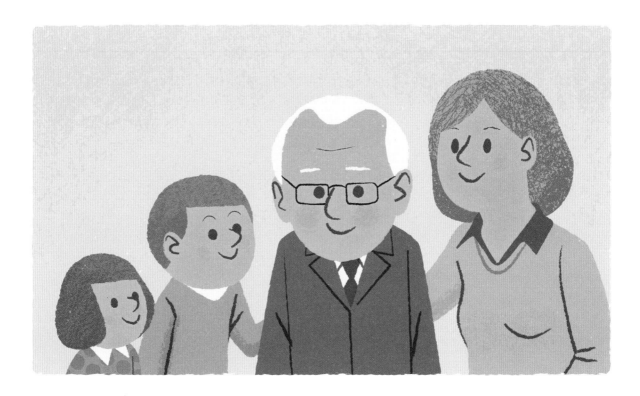

When the war ended, Captain Tom left the army and built a family, but he never forgot his friends. He started a reunion dinner that went on for 65 long years, until finally, it was just him answering his own invitation.

He was 90 when he slipped during his daily walk. After a few visits to the hospital, Captain Tom left with a ton of gratitude for the nurses and doctors who took care of him. And also, with a hip replacement and two new knees.

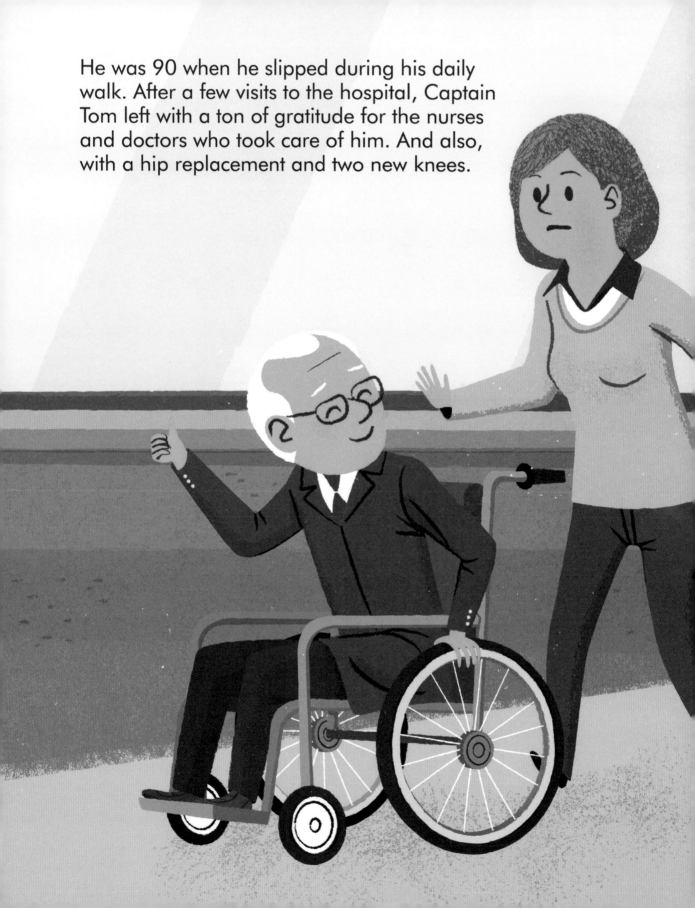

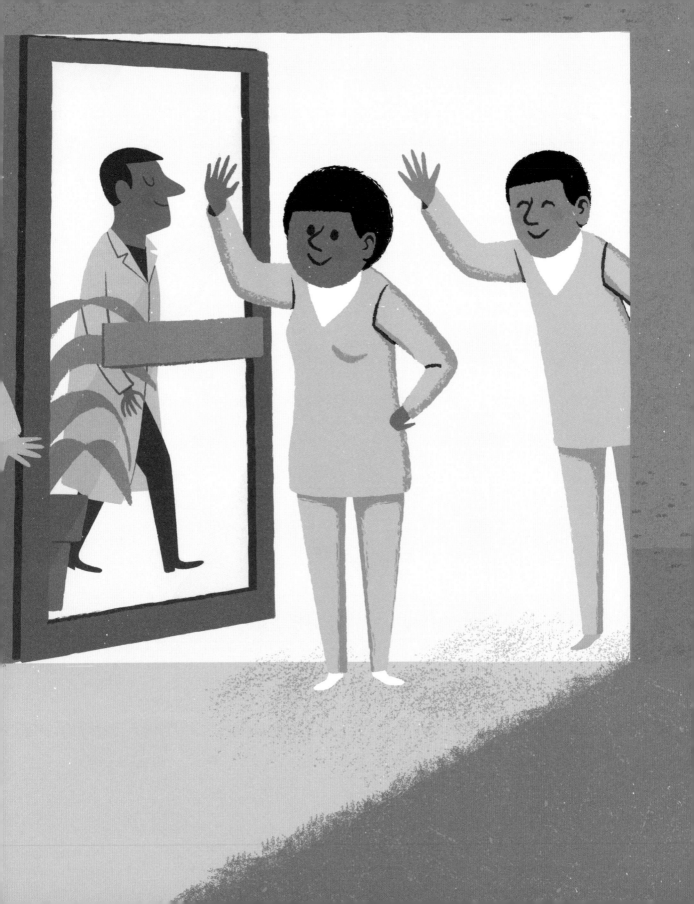

It takes just one step after another to get well, and Captain Tom couldn't wait to take the first. When his daughter found a treadmill on the drive and discovered it was Grandpa Tom who had bought it online, she felt very proud of him.

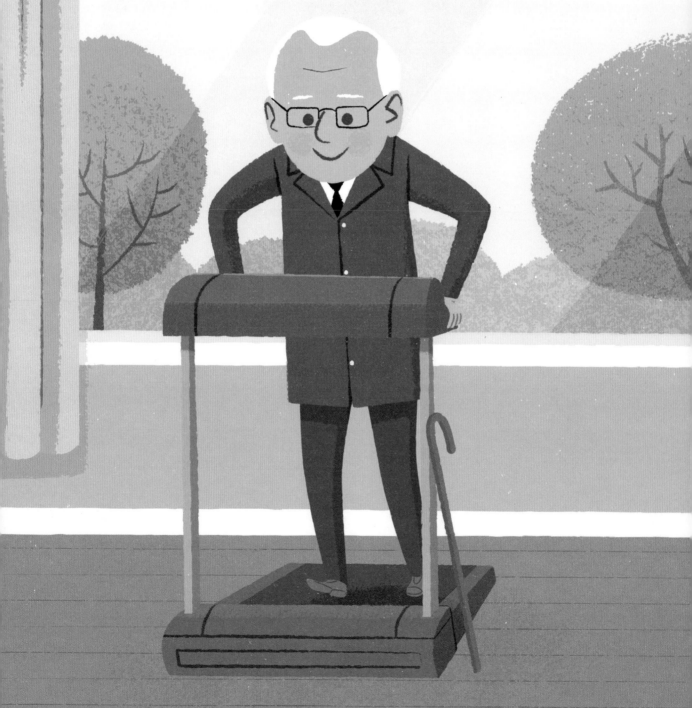

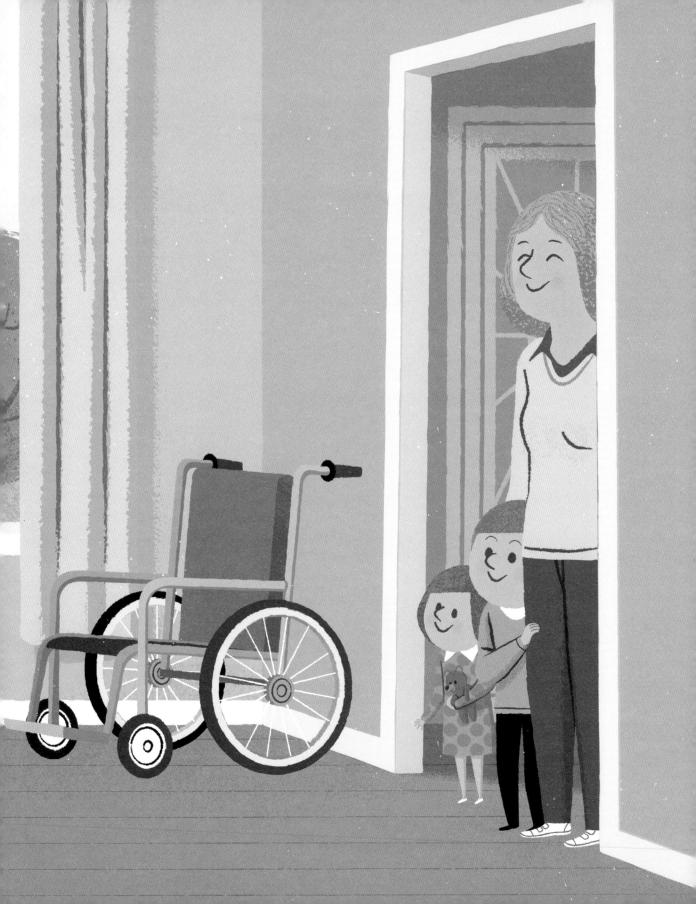

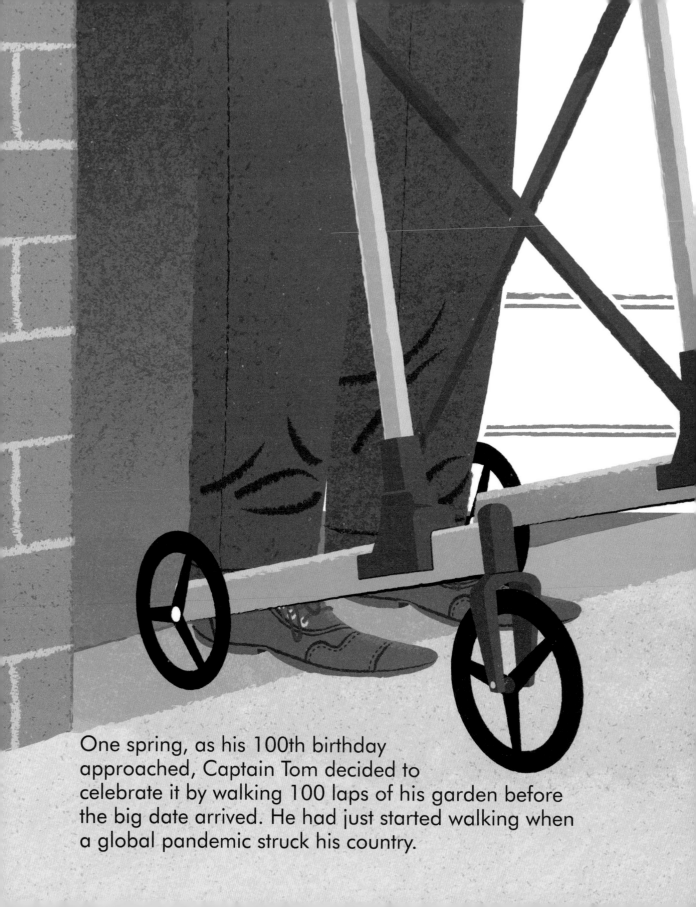

One spring, as his 100th birthday approached, Captain Tom decided to celebrate it by walking 100 laps of his garden before the big date arrived. He had just started walking when a global pandemic struck his country.

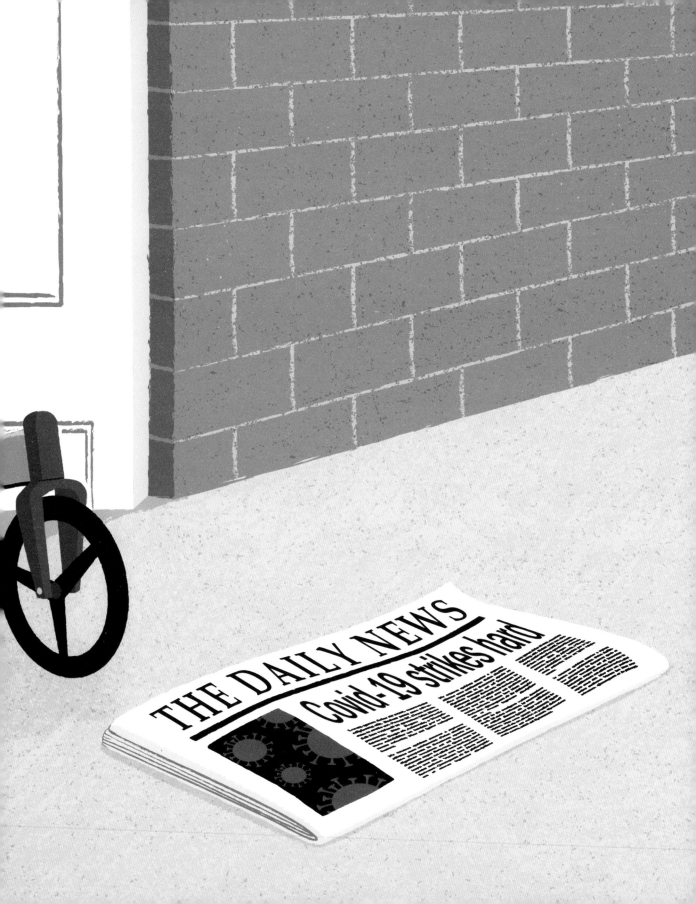

Holding his walking frame even tighter, Captain Tom kept marching with a new goal in mind. To raise one thousand pounds for those who once took care of him, and now were on the front line helping others: the healthcare staff.

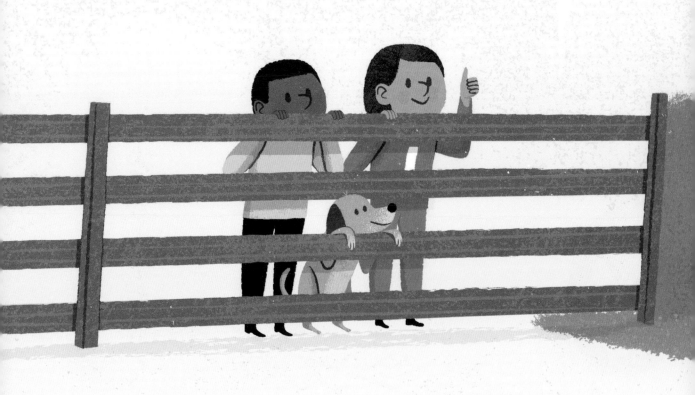

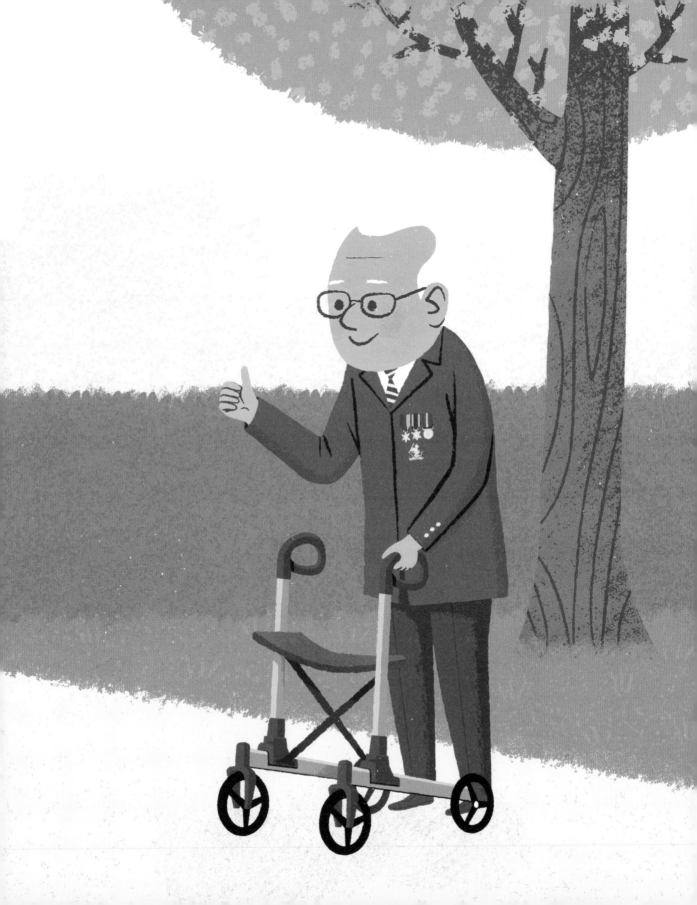

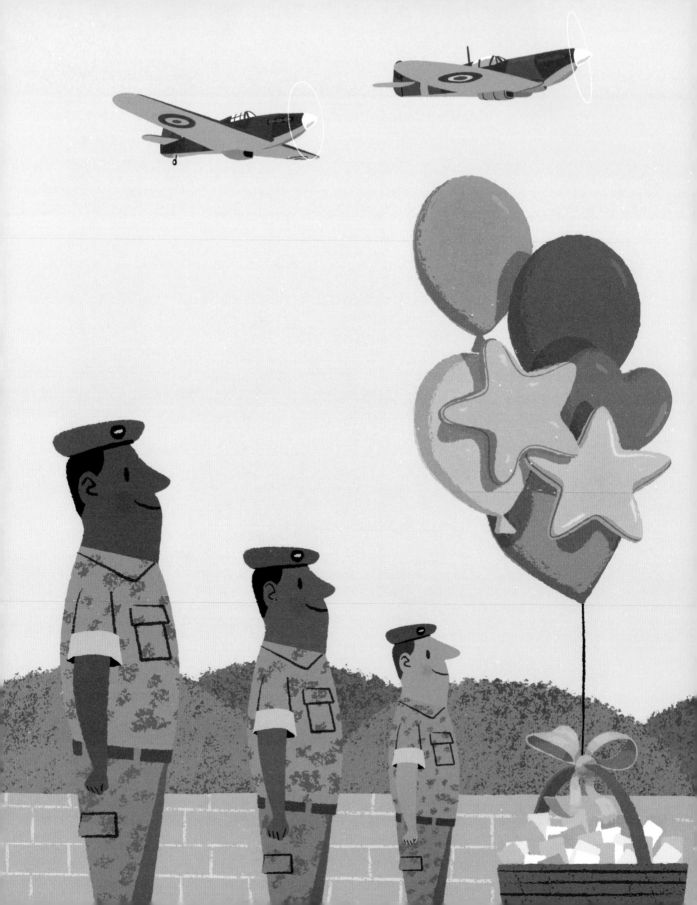

Everyone was so touched by Captain Tom's feat that, by his birthday, he raised more than 30 million pounds! His regiment was there to salute him, and he was sent cards from people all over the country, even from the Queen.

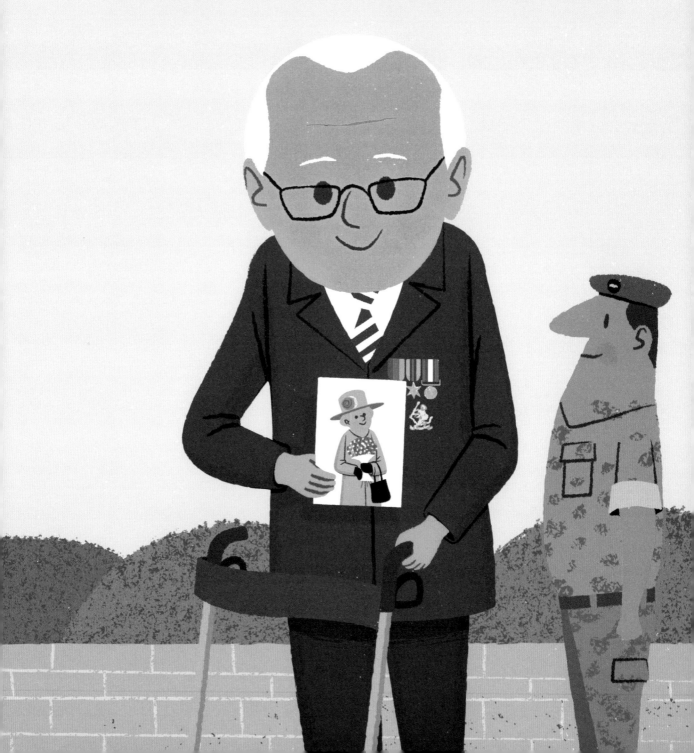

And tomorrow will be a new day and the sun will shine, as little Tom goes for his daily stroll. The humble hero and national treasure, who invites us to keep walking next to him, never leaving anyone behind.

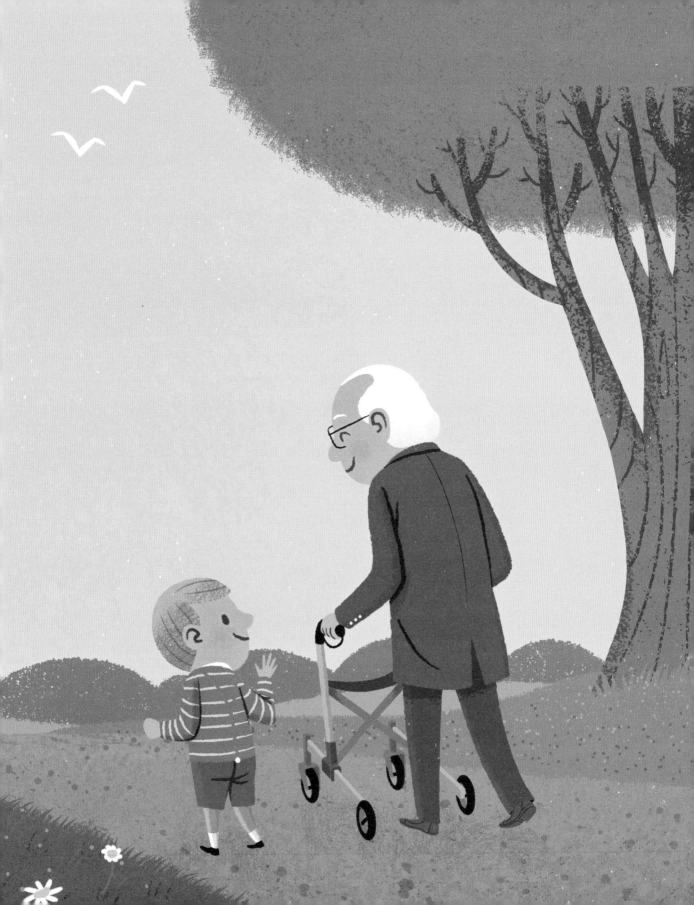

CAPTAIN TOM

(Born 1920)

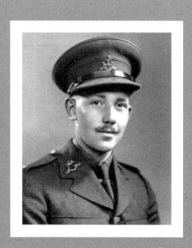

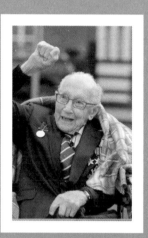

c. 1940

2020

Tom Moore was born in Yorkshire in 1920. The world had just recovered from a flu pandemic, and people were starting to rebuild. Tom grew up with a love for all things practical and a knack for finding something to do to help. By the time Tom was 20, he was on his way to becoming a civil engineer. But then the world changed as another crisis struck: World War Two. In the army, Tom was sent to India, Burma and Sumatra, where he helped keep tanks chugging along, and eventually was promoted to Captain. After the war, there was more rebuilding to do. The UK's National Health Service (NHS) was set up, which makes sure that people can get free healthcare at the point of use. Tom went back to Yorkshire, swapping tanks for motorcycles, which he raced and repaired. He married and raised

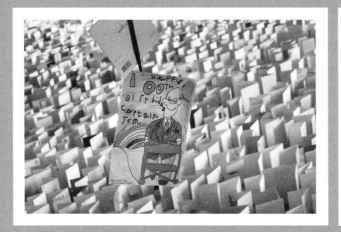

2020

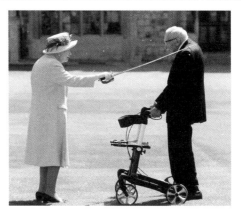

2020

a family, living a quiet, happy life. But when Tom was 99, a pandemic hit, caused by the coronavirus. People were asked to stay at home to stop the spread and protect everyone's health. But trust Captain Tom to find something to do to help! In his army uniform and supported by his walking frame, he aimed to raise £1,000 for the NHS by walking 100 laps of his garden by his 100th birthday. Soon, people across the world were inspired by his goal, and had donated over £30 million! His 100th lap was celebrated with an RAF flyover, an honorary promotion to Colonel, and 120,000 birthday cards from people in the UK and beyond. He was even knighted by the Queen! Captain Sir Tom Moore shows the world that the best way to rebuild after a crisis is to come together – and keep on walking.

Want to find out more about **Captain Tom?**

Have a read of these great books:

One Hundred Steps: The Story of Captain Sir Tom Moore

by Captain Tom Moore and Adam Larkum

Brimming with creative inspiration, how-to projects, and useful information to enrich your everyday life, Quarto Knows is a favourite destination for those pursuing their interests and passions. Visit our site and dig deeper with our books into your area of interest: Quarto Creates, Quarto Cooks, Quarto Homes, Quarto Lives, Quarto Drives, Quarto Explores, Quarto Gifts, or Quarto Kids.

Text © 2020 Maria Isabel Sánchez Vegara. Illustrations © Christophe Jacques 2020.
Original concept of the series by Maria Isabel Sánchez Vegara, published by Alba Editorial, s.l.u
Produced under licence from Alba Editorial s.l.u and Beautifool Couple S.L.
First Published in the UK in 2020 by Frances Lincoln Children's Books, an imprint of The Quarto Group.
The Old Brewery, 6 Blundell Street, London N7 9BH, United Kingdom.
T 020 7700 6700 **www.QuartoKnows.com**

A catalogue record for this book is available from the British Library.
ISBN 978-0-7112-6207-2
Set in Futura BT.

Published by Katie Cotton • Designed by Karissa Santos
Edited by Katy Flint • Production by Nikki Ingram
Editorial Assistance from Alex Hithersay
Manufactured in Guangdong, China CC112020
3 5 7 9 8 6 4

Photographic acknowledgements (pages 28-29, from left to right): 1. Tom Moore (soldier), c. 1940, public domain. 2. Tom Moore, Military Veteran Who Raised Funds For NHS, Celebrates 100th Birthday, 2020 © Emma Sohl – Capture the Light Photography via Getty Images. 3. Birthday cards sent to Captain Tom Moore for his 100th birthday © Photo by Shaun Botterill/Getty. 4. Britain's Queen Elizabeth II uses the sword that belonged to her father, George VI as she confers the Honour of Knighthood on 100-year-old veteran Captain Tom Moore at Windsor Castle in Windsor, west of London on July 17, 2020 © Photo by CHRIS JACKSON/POOL/AFP via Getty Images.

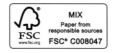

Collect the *Little People,* **BIG DREAMS**® series:

FRIDA KAHLO
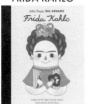
ISBN: 978-1-84780-770-0

COCO CHANEL
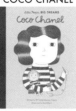
ISBN: 978-1-84780-771-7

MAYA ANGELOU

ISBN: 978-1-84780-890-5

AMELIA EARHART
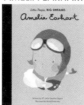
ISBN: 978-1-84780-885-1

AGATHA CHRISTIE
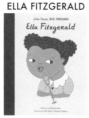
ISBN: 978-1-84780-959-9

MARIE CURIE
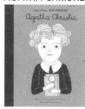
ISBN: 978-1-84780-961-2

ROSA PARKS
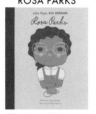
ISBN: 978-1-78603-017-7

AUDREY HEPBURN
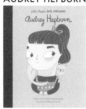
ISBN: 978-1-78603-052-8

EMMELINE PANKHURST
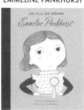
ISBN: 978-1-78603-019-1

ELLA FITZGERALD
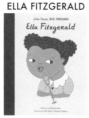
ISBN: 978-1-78603-086-3

ADA LOVELACE
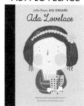
ISBN: 978-1-78603-075-7

JANE AUSTEN
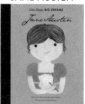
ISBN: 978-1-78603-119-8

GEORGIA O'KEEFFE
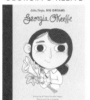
ISBN: 978-1-78603-121-1

HARRIET TUBMAN
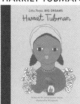
ISBN: 978-1-78603-289-8

ANNE FRANK
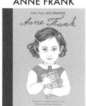
ISBN: 978-1-78603-292-8

MOTHER TERESA
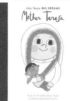
ISBN: 978-1-78603-290-4

JOSEPHINE BAKER
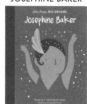
ISBN: 978-1-78603-291-1

L. M. MONTGOMERY
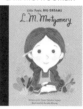
ISBN: 978-1-78603-295-9

JANE GOODALL
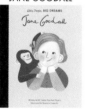
ISBN: 978-1-78603-294-2

SIMONE DE BEAUVOIR
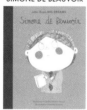
ISBN: 978-1-78603-293-5

MUHAMMAD ALI
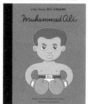
ISBN: 978-1-78603-733-6

STEPHEN HAWKING
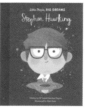
ISBN: 978-1-78603-732-9

MARIA MONTESSORI
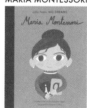
ISBN: 978-1-78603-753-4

VIVIENNE WESTWOOD
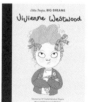
ISBN: 978-1-78603-756-5

MAHATMA GANDHI
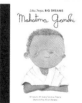
ISBN: 978-1-78603-334-5

DAVID BOWIE
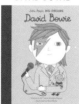
ISBN: 978-1-78603-803-6

WILMA RUDOLPH
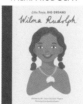
ISBN: 978-1-78603-750-3

DOLLY PARTON
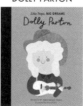
ISBN: 978-1-78603-759-6

BRUCE LEE
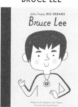
ISBN: 978-1-78603-335-2

RUDOLF NUREYEV
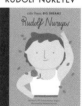
ISBN: 978-1-78603-336-9

ZAHA HADID
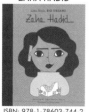
ISBN: 978-1-78603-744-2

MARY SHELLEY
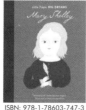
ISBN: 978-1-78603-747-3

MARTIN LUTHER KING JR.
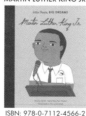
ISBN: 978-0-7112-4566-2

DAVID ATTENBOROUGH
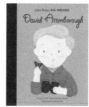
ISBN: 978-0-7112-4563-1

ASTRID LINDGREN
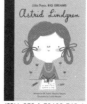
ISBN: 978-1-78603-762-6

EVONNE GOOLAGONG
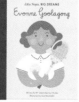
ISBN: 978-0-7112-4585-3

BOB DYLAN
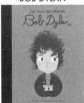
ISBN: 978-0-7112-4674-4

ALAN TURING
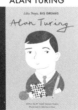
ISBN: 978-0-7112-4677-5

BILLIE JEAN KING
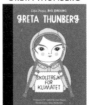
ISBN: 978-0-7112-4692-8

GRETA THUNBERG
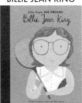
ISBN: 978-0-7112-5643-9

JESSE OWENS
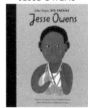
ISBN: 978-0-7112-4582-2

JEAN-MICHEL BASQUIAT
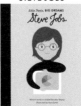
ISBN: 978-0-7112-4579-2

ARETHA FRANKLIN
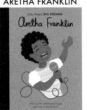
ISBN: 978-0-7112-4687-4

CORAZON AQUINO
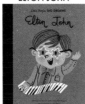
ISBN: 978-0-7112-4683-6

PELÉ
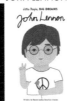
ISBN: 978-0-7112-4574-7

ERNEST SHACKLETON
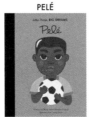
ISBN: 978-0-7112-4570-9

STEVE JOBS
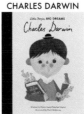
ISBN: 978-0-7112-4576-1

AYRTON SENNA
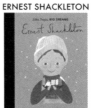
ISBN: 978-0-7112-4671-3

LOUISE BOURGEOIS
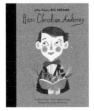
ISBN: 978-0-7112-4689-8

ELTON JOHN
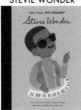
ISBN: 978-0-7112-5838-9

JOHN LENNON
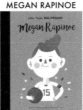
ISBN: 978-0-7112-5765-8

PRINCE
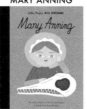
ISBN: 978-0-7112-5437-4

CHARLES DARWIN
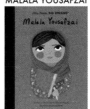
ISBN: 978-0-7112-5769-6

CAPTAIN TOM MOORE
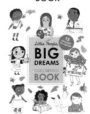
ISBN: 978-0-7112-6207-2

HANS CHRISTIAN ANDERSEN
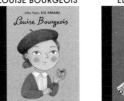
ISBN: 978-0-7112-5932-4

STEVIE WONDER
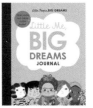
ISBN: 978-0-7112-5773-3

MEGAN RAPINOE
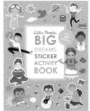
ISBN: 978-0-7112-5781-8

MARY ANNING
ISBN: 978-0-7112-5551-7

MALALA YOUSAFZAI
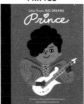
ISBN: 978-0-7112-5902-7

ACTIVITY BOOKS

STICKER ACTIVITY BOOK
ISBN: 978-0-7112-6011-5

COLOURING BOOK
ISBN: 978-0-7112-6135-8

LITTLE ME, BIG DREAMS JOURNAL
ISBN: 978-0-7112-4888-5

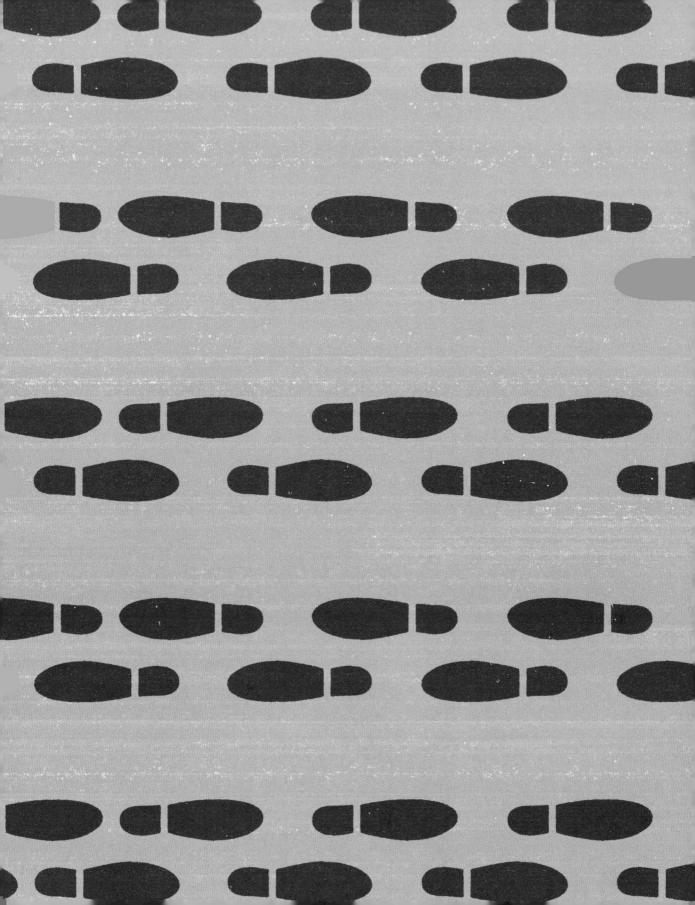